HOW TO QUIT SMOKING:

A QUICK GUIDE TO FREE YOUR MIND AND BODY FROM NICOTINE ADDICTION AND TO STOP SMOKING CIGARETTES

J.C. Gunlee

I0412328

i

TABLE OF CONTENTS

1   Introduction

"The secret of getting ahead is getting started." Mark Twain

Life is hard. That is a truth. But quitting smoking does not have to be hard. It can be and should be an enjoyable experience. I can tell you from a first-hand experience that quitting smoking can be enjoyable. Like most (or perhaps all) people who are reading this, I used to be addicted to cigarettes. I had been chained to the slavery that is cigarette smoking for over twenty years. While I'm neither a doctor nor a therapist, I believe my experience as a former confirmed smoker provides me with a much more applicable experience than one that can be provided by any formal education. I used to think that life could never really be as enjoyable without cigarettes. Like most smokers, I tried many times to quit smoking during those years. Sometimes succeeding ... from several days at a time to several months. But ultimately, my so-called "will power" caved, and I took a drag of the nicotine stick, and I was back at it again. Except the last time. My former thinking that I could not enjoy life without cigarettes was completely off the mark. Now I know that life is much more enjoyable without cigarettes, not only because I know that I'm healthier now, but because I now understand clearly that cigarettes never provided any benefits to me while I was using them. Since quitting smoking for good years ago, I can honestly say that I have never felt the urge to smoke a cigarette. What made the difference? It is in the frame of mind and the clarity of the relevant issues.

This book is not a monumental compendium of all the facts and techniques for quitting smoking, but merely a short synopsis on the techniques and ideas that I have used to successfully quit smoking for good. You may be reading this because you truly want to kick the habit, or may be because someone who loves you put you up to quitting smoking. Whatever the reason is for your decision to pick up this book, you owe it to yourself to follow through and finish. After all,

you have nothing to lose and everything to gain.

2   Recognize that you are a nicotine addict.

"Expect problems and eat them for breakfast." Alfred

Montapert

The first step in solving a problem is to recognize that there is a problem. By picking up this book, you probably realize that there is an issue, and you are trying to work your way to address the issue. You have to be clear about what that issue is, and with respect to what we are talking about here, the issue that you have to recognize is that you are addicted to the nicotine stick called cigarette.

What does it mean to be addicted to nicotine? It means that you may have a strong urge to smoke when you drink a cup of coffee. Or when you have a beer, some liquor, or a cocktail. Or right after you have a meal. Or when you use the restroom for the #2. Or when you wake up in the morning. Or before you brush your teeth at night. Or when you are stressed. Or when you are out with friends. Or any number of other "triggers." Or when there is no "trigger" at all. Or when you are simply bored. Simply put, if you have the urge to get a hold of that little nicotine stick called cigarette habitually, you have an addiction to that nicotine smoke stick.

Some smokers think that they are not addicts because they may not be smoking on a daily basis. They may be a weekend-smoker or smoke only when they "go out." If you are one of these people, think about why you smoke, and whether you can truly "take it or leave it." If you think you can stop it and do without the smokes, then simply go ahead and stop smoking. If you can do this—if you can stop smoking for good without any further thought or guidance—then good for you, you are not an addict. You do not need this book, and you should stop smoking now. For if you continue to smoke even only a few times a month, you will certainly become an addict. It may take a pack of cigarettes or it may take a hundred, and it may take a few weeks after your first cigarette or it may take several years, but sooner or later, the nicotine beggar will establish its presence inside you and you will be hooked. As you smoke more, you are feeding the nicotine beggar, and your tolerance for nicotine will increase. The nicotine beggar will demand more from you, and you will need to get your fix more regularly. That is the nature of an addiction. It grows on you, and your mind and body will readjust to serve its new and growing master—your addiction. Soon enough, you might smoke a few per day, which could turn into a half a pack, then a pack a day, and may be even more. And, as virtually all smokers do at one time or another, you will regret the day that you first started smoking.

Smokers are addicts, and addicts are often times too clever with themselves in trying to deceive their own mind. This is because smokers are rational people, and would like to think of themselves as reasonable human beings in the face of the undeniable fact they know deep inside—that smoking is killing them. They rationalize their purported "choice" to smoke cigarettes. This is ultimately a mind trick, denials, and excuses to continue the feeding of their nicotine addiction. Now, fifty years after the release of the first Surgeon General's report warning of the health hazards of smoking, nobody can deny that smoking is toxic and highly addictive, and that nicotine is the drug and the primary substance in a cigarette causing the addiction. Smokers may create rationalization in their mind that they enjoy smoking, or that smoking relaxes them or provides other "benefits." Smokers rarely think these purported "benefits" through. But if they do, they will find that their alleged reasons for smoking are merely false rationalizations. It is the nicotine beggar inside you that is conjuring up rationalizations to continue such destructive behavior that harms your mind and body.

Addicts may also avoid thinking about why they smoke, often because they do not want to face the truth about their addiction problems. They may say to themselves

"Today is not a good day to quit; perhaps tomorrow or the next week; perhaps when I don't have so much stuff to do; perhaps when this stressful situation is over; perhaps after the party this weekend." Set aside such tendencies and recognize your addiction now. There is no better time to start than today. You will find that you can dismantle your addiction easier if you confront it head on now.

3   An addict's mind is riddled with internal conflicts.

"If you're going through hell, keep going." Winston Churchill

Addiction requires an action. Addiction is an obsession about something and acting on that obsession. This behavior limits the addicted person's freedom within his or her own mind and body. Addiction strains your inner psyche by pulling your will—your capacity to make choices—in two opposite directions. One part of your mind wants to be free from your addiction, while the other part wants to continue feeding it. This internal conflict is a battle that a smoker engages in constantly. Smokers deal with such conflicts by fooling and deceiving themselves. They might say to themselves, "I'm an adult, and I choose to smoke through my own free will; smoking is not all that bad for my health, and besides, I don't care to live 'till I'm 100 anyways, and my cigarette is my friend in need when I'm stressed and need a break." They create elaborate excuses and rationales to belittle or ignore the detrimental effects of smoking while embellishing the purported "benefit" of smoking. All of these are mind tricks that an addict creates for one single purpose: to keep the nicotine addiction going.

The internal conflict that an addiction creates in a person's willpower also hurts the person's self-esteem. For instance, when smokers try to kick the habit and fail (and virtually all smokers have failed at quitting at one time or another), such a failure erodes the smoker's self-esteem. Indeed, it would be difficult not to feel defeated about such a failure. The smoker would feel a loss of self-control, shame, guilt, and remorse. If I cannot make myself act according to my own willpower, how am I better than a slave beholden to a master? To deal with such degradation in self-esteem, the smoker might repress the failure, or might deny that there was any failure, or might create more rationalizations and mind tricks. Perhaps the smoker might say to himself "I did not really want to quit anyways; I'll quit next year; next year will not be too late; besides, I like smoking; it helps me cope with life." Again, these excuses and rationalizations have only one purpose: to keep feeding the nicotine beggar inside the smoker.

A human mind is clever and will constantly invent new ways to further an addiction. One subtle way to this end is trying to delay addressing the problem. An addict's mind might suggest that "Let's not rush into this important step of quitting smoking; I need to really think deeply about the strategies, plans, and reasons for quitting." Such a delay tactic might often work, and the addict can simply forget about quitting for a while, until the addict remembers that he or she had planned to quit. Then the delay can happen again. Or the addict can come up with numerous other tactics to quit, such as waiting for that "perfect" time to quit, perhaps it's on New Years Day, or an anniversary date, or his or her birthday, or perhaps a religiously significant date, or some other date. There is no need to set such an arbitrary date. The time for quitting is now, and there is no need to complicate the process of quitting smoking. You do not need to set aside weeks, days, or even hours in order for you to quit. Quitting smoking does not take a lot of time; it may even save you time, as you no longer would need to waste time poisoning yourself several times a day with cigarette smoke.

It is said that suffering is caused by attachments.[1] This truth cannot be more appropriate in the context of an addiction, as a nicotine addiction is indeed an attachment that causes suffering in every aspect of your mind and body. It is important to examine the nature of the attachment that you have for a cigarette. Understanding the nature of your attachment is an important step towards achieving freedom from your addiction.

---

[1] This is one of the "Four Noble Truths" in Buddhist teachings.

4   Smoking does not relieve stress or provide relaxation.

"With the new day comes new strength and new thoughts." Eleanor Roosevelt

May be you keep smoking because you think it relaxes you. But, as you might already know, nicotine is a stimulant—a category of drugs that is opposite of relaxation. Smoking does not "calm your nerves" or relax you. Rather, cigarette raises your blood pressure and heart rate. The nicotine kick is quick. And that is the primary reason why nicotine is such an effective addiction mechanism. Nicotine also leaves the body quickly, which prompts further urges to get more of it. And you smoke more to get more nicotine, which prompts further urges, and the cycle continues. Once you accept what smoking and nicotine is doing to you, you can come to an understanding that the only stress that a cigarette is relieving is the stress that is generated from the urge for the lack of nicotine.

If smoking actually relieves external stress and achieves relaxation, smokers would be the most relaxed and stress-free people in the world. But do you think that is true or even plausible? The opposite is true. Smokers are some of the most stressed out and agitated people. Once you accept your nicotine addiction, the reason for the smoker's irritability and tenseness is obvious. Once the effects of nicotine wears off—which is quick—the smoker has the urges to smoke more. And when a smoker cannot have another smoke for the time being, that creates the stress. The stress for more nicotine. There may be many occasions to bring about such a stress. Indeed, smokers spend most of their lives in places where they cannot smoke. May be you are at a park that does not allow smoking. Or you are at work waiting for that "smoke break." Or you are in a restaurant, which undoubtedly is non-smoking in these days. Or you are in an airplane. Or you are with family who does not want you to smoke (or does not know that you smoke).

Smokers in these situations are tense, in a sense of panic, and often cannot think of anything other than to scope out the next opportunity to feed their addiction. And imagine the panic that smokers feel when they are out of cigarettes late at night and "need" to smoke. Nonsmokers do not have to feel this panic or stress. Realize that it is the cigarette itself that creates and perpetuates the stress. By having a cigarette, you are guaranteeing to have the stress of worrying about the next smoking opportunity. Your addiction to cigarette adds stress to an otherwise pleasant walk in the park, and exacerbates your stress levels in situations that are already stressful, such as an important meeting.

And what happens when you light that cancer stick in your mouth? If you were like me, you would immediately regret lighting it up and ask yourself "Why am I smoking?" Cigarette addiction is in a way unlike many other addictions. Cigarette is desirable only when you cannot have it, and it immediately ceases being desirable the moment you actually taste it. Lighting that cigarette merely relieves the tension that was created by the last nicotine stick that you have sucked on. It merely feeds the nicotine beggar inside you, but just for a little while, and the vicious cycle continues with your next cigarette, and on and on. Smokers often confuse the relief they get from a cigarette. Smoking does not relieve any stress that is not caused by the cigarette itself. For example, the stress that you might have had from that big meeting you have in an hour is still there, if not exacerbated by the rise in blood pressure resulting from the nicotine. At the same time, smoking generates the urges for more nicotine in the future, causing further stressful situations to come in the near future. Indeed, some people try to pre-empt such situations by becoming chain smokers. Chain smokers are some of the most stress-ridden people in the world. And make no mistake about it: smoking is contributing to the stress—and likely the primary cause of stress—in chain smokers.

Some smokers have also created a rationalization in their mind that smoking helps them concentrate. This is merely another mind trick conjured up by the nicotine beggar inside them. Smoking cannot provide you with better concentration for the same reason that it does not relieve stress. It is indeed difficult to concentrate better when you have to mind the cigarette beggar begging you to feed it more nicotine. Nonsmokers do not need to worry about such things. And think about the act of smoking. First, you often have to go out of your way to find a place where you can smoke and hold a burning object in your hand for several minutes at a time many times a day, interrupting whatever you were doing. Smoking is nothing but a distraction to whatever you want to concentrate on.

Aside from the stress created by the nicotine addiction, there may be stress that is caused by external circumstances resulting from cigarette smoking. Smoking in public places—like restaurants, bars, workplaces, and parks—are becoming less and less common, due in part to cities and other government entities passing laws prohibiting smoking in certain places. This is also due in part to decades of public education that has rightfully informed the public that smoking is harmful not only to the smoker but also to everyone around the smoker, due to secondhand smoke. While smoking may have been widely accepted socially in the distant past, those days are long gone. Smoking is undoubtedly an antisocial activity in the modern world. Have you ever been on the receiving end of those disapproving eyes from friends or strangers when you took out a cigarette to smoke in a public place? This happens even in places where smoking is not prohibited. But who can blame them—you are putting nonsmoker's health at risk through secondhand smoke coming from your cigarette.

Stress can come also from the fact that you have friends, family, or loved ones that want you to quit smoking. If you are like me, you may have even promised your spouse or significant other that you will not smoke. And I am ashamed to admit that countless times I have broken that promise. Sometimes I have tried to hide from my wife the fact that I have smoked, by smoking in secret, and then brushing my teeth and washing my hands. That tactic has never really worked, as my wife has a nose like a bloodhound, and it is difficult to wipe clean the nasty cigarette smell in your mouth, tongue, fingers, and hair. I have always dreaded disappointing my wife that I have broken my promise to stop smoking. But even in the face of such a stress, I had often given in to my addiction and acted to feed the nicotine beggar inside me. I felt like a fraud and a criminal, smoking in secret from my wife, afraid whether she would find out that I smoked, afraid that she would find the cigarettes I had hidden in the garage. Nonsmokers do not have to worry about whether others can smell the rotten cigarette on you or whether others can see the black and brown stains on your teeth. Nonsmokers similarly do not have to worry about all the complications in interpersonal relationships that arise because of your vile addiction to nicotine.

Such is the nature of cigarette addiction—it causes stress inside you through your physical and mental addiction to the substance, and it causes stress externally through your personal relationships and with the public at large. The notion that a cigarette "relaxes" you is a myth created by a smoker's mind to rationalize the nicotine addiction. Do not fall for this mind trick.

5 Withdrawal symptom is virtually all in your mind and is short-lived.

"Start where you are. Use what you have. Do what you can." Arthur Ashe

Some smokers are afraid to quit because of the alleged "withdrawal" symptoms that they may experience. There is nothing to be scared of. Although you may be irritable and experience some urges to smoke, you will be fine. Indeed, the irritability and urges to smoke exist in days when you are continuing to smoke. Withdrawal from nicotine is all in your head after a day or two of stopping smoking. For instance, have you ever heard of anyone dying from nicotine withdrawal? Me neither. As bad as you may think the purported "withdrawal" is at times, it will not kill you. It will not even come close. All you may feel is a little irritation. Think about why you feel the irritation—it is the nicotine beggar inside you that is pleading for a hit of nicotine smoke. It has no power over you other than what you grant it; it will not make you sick; it will not make you vomit; it will not disable you or make you unable to walk. In fact, the withdrawal is the same irritation that smokers go through everyday. In fact, it is this withdrawal irritation that is the primary driver that fuels the addiction. Most smokers can go smoke-free for hours at a time even with this physical withdrawal symptom. Indeed, virtually all smokers sleep through the night in withdrawal, and the withdrawal symptom does not bother them enough to wake them up.

Will smoking a cigarette make your withdrawal symptom and urge go away? Yes, that is the nature of the nicotine addiction, or any drug addiction for that matter. But it is merely temporary. And it is crucial to remember that the withdrawal symptoms are **created** by the cigarette. In other words, you will never get rid of the withdrawal symptom if you continue to smoke. Cigarettes do not provide true relief from withdrawal. They are the poison that causes the withdrawal in the first place, and they perpetuate your withdrawal symptoms as long as you keep smoking.

Nicotine is a fast acting substance, both in terms of it going inside your body and coming out of your system. Nicotine level drops almost immediately after you put out your cigarette. After seven or eight hours after your last cigarette, more than 90% of nicotine is out of your system. Nicotine typically leaves a smoker's bloodstream completely within 1-3 days. In other words, after that first 1 to 3 days, everything is purely psychological. It is all in your head. And, during those first few days, the physiological symptoms merely amounts to some urges or pangs that you feel when you are hungry, except that your nicotine beggar inside you is hungry for a nicotine hit, rather than your stomach longing for nutritious food. Nicotine withdrawal does not cause physical pain. Withdrawal is merely a temporary restlessness, a mild irritation. For those first few days, you can fight the urges through various distractions that you can employ, such as watching some TV or a movie, reading a book, surfing the web, playing with your dog or cat, working, catching some sleep, or doing your favorite hobby.

After those first few days, any urges that you feel will not be a physiological reaction. It is all mental. This is not to say that mental urges are any less powerful than physical urges. But it might be comforting knowing that the urge you feel after those first few days is literally all in your mind. You will still think about smoking and have mental urge to smoke, particularly relating to your "trigger" situations, such as with a coffee or beer, after a meal, in the bathroom, etc. It is important to realize that these are merely psychological, and its effect is only as big as you make it out to be. What you do with your mental urges is all up to you, and you will suffer no physical effects by simply saying "no" to a cigarette. Think of this phase as a situation where you moved into a new place to live. For a first few days, or perhaps a couple of weeks, you will not feel "at home" in your new place. But soon enough, you will get used to your new room and house, and things will feel natural and at home. Similarly, you are mind and body will not feel "at home" in your new life as a non-smoker for a few days, but soon enough, not smoking will come naturally, even when a "trigger" situation presents itself.

6   Focus on the benefits of smoking (hint: there are no benefits).

"The pessimist complains about the wind; the optimist expects it to change; the realist adjusts the sails." William

Arthur Ward

People who try to quit often focus on the benefits of not smoking or the harms of smoking, which is a different side of the same coin. But that is not where the focus should be when you are trying to quit.   The focus should be squarely on thinking about and understanding the **benefits of smoking**, or the lack thereof.   Give yourself a few moments or a day to think about what you believe are the benefits of smoking—I mean really think about it.

There are many things that a smoker could come up with as the purported "benefits" that he or she gets in smoking.   One of the most common things smokers say when asked why they smoke is "smoking relaxes me" or "smoking relieves my stress." But, as you know, nicotine is a stimulant. Smoking raises your heart rate and blood pressure. It makes you "wired," albeit in mild and ineffective manner.

A smoker may still insist that smoking provides "relaxation" or "relief" from stress, but the smoker may be misattributing the effects of the cigarette smoke with his or her smoking routine. For example, the routine of going on a "smoke break" may actually provide relaxation or stress relief, but that's not from the nicotine stick. Rather, the relaxation comes from the fact that the smoker is on a break. Next time you want to take a "smoke break," by all means, go for a break, but without smoking. Instead, go outside and take a deep breath. Even in the most polluted of cities, a deep breath of air outside will be more refreshing and relaxing than taking a puff of the toxic, carcinogenic cigarette smoke.

Like in a "smoke break," a form of relaxation may come from situations in which smokers find themselves when they are smoking, but they are giving the undeserved credit to the cigarette smoke. This applies to virtually every "trigger" situations. If one of your trigger situation is going #2 in the bathroom, that situation relieves stress certainly—but the relief is coming by way of (or into) the toilet, not by way of cigarette smoke going into your mouth, throat, and lungs.

Also remember that the supposed "stress" to be relieved is created by smoking cigarettes. Smokers are stressed when they want to smoke but cannot, for one reason or another. The time for the meeting to end, or the "smoke break" to come, or the class to finish, or the flight to land, or numerous other non-smoking situation to end cannot come soon enough for devoted smokers, so that they can go outside, take out their cancer sticks, and take a puff to feed the nicotine beggar inside them. Such situations create tremendous stress in smokers—stress that nonsmokers never have to face. Nonsmokers are not antsy to go outside in freezing or raining weather to take a puff of toxic smoke.

Smoking provides neither relaxation nor relief from stress. If you believe there are any benefits to smoking, give it some thought and think about the reasons. You will soon come to an understanding that you smoke because you are addicted to the nicotine smoke, and not because there are any benefits to smoking. It is very important that you come to this understanding—that you truly know in your heart and mind that there are no benefits to smoking. A cigarette is not your stress reliever, a relaxation aid, or your "friend." A cigarette is simply a cancer stick that you have been duped into taking day-in-and-day-out because you have been conditioned to do so over time, and re-enforced to do so through the nicotine chemical in the cigarette. The act of smoking is a disease, disease of the mind. Accept this fact. Once you accept this truth, stopping smoking becomes easy.

7   Nicotine and other toxic chemicals are in cigarette smoke.

"Start wide, expand further, and never look back." Arnold

Schwarzenegger

Nicotine is the primary chemical that causes addiction to cigarettes. Nicotine's immediate toxicity is dependent on how much you take it, how long and how often you have taken it, the way nicotine has been received (e.g., through inhaling, chewing, ingesting, etc.), formulation of the nicotine product, among other things. Some symptoms of toxicity include nausea and vomiting, to diarrhea, and increased salivation. More severe dosage can lead to seizures and respiratory pressures. *See* The Health Consequences of Smoking—50 Years of Progress, A Report of the Surgeon General, U.S. Dept. of Health & Human Services (2014) at 111. Numerous nicotine poisoning has been documented since the use of nicotine as a pesticide became widespread in the earlier part of the twentieth century. *Id.* at 112.

People have died from nicotine poisoning. *Id.*

Nicotine has significant risks for pregnancies, babies, and children. There is experimental evidence to conclude that nicotine causes premature births and stillbirths. *See* The Health Consequences of Smoking—50 Years of Progress, A Report of the Surgeon General, U.S. Dept. of Health & Human Services (2014) at 126. Nicotine exposure also causes lasting harm to brain development in babies and adolescents. While more studies need to be conducted to establish a definite link between nicotine and cancer, there is sufficient evidence to conclude that nicotine increases the risks for multiple diseases, such as cardiovascular and lung diseases. *See id.* at 126. The detrimental effect of nicotine is not surprising. Nicotine is a well known poison, and has been widely used in insecticides, particularly in the past, *e.g.,* in the 1950s and 60s. The use of nicotine in insecticides has declined in recent years due to the fact that there are insecticides that are cheaper and less harmful to mammals. These days, nicotine is prohibited as a pesticide for organic farming in the United States.

It is also important to remember that nicotine is but one chemical in a cigarette stick. There more than 250 chemicals in tobacco smoke that are known to be detrimental to health, including hydrogen cyanide, carbon monoxide, ammonia, arsenic, benzene, beryllium (a toxic metal), 1,3–butadiene (a hazardous gas), cadmium (a toxic metal), chromium, ethylene oxide, polonium-210 (a radioactive chemical element), vinyl chloride, formaldehyde, benzo pyrene, toluene, and others. These chemicals are known or suspected to cause cancer and other deadly diseases.

8   Admit that a cigarette tastes nasty.

"By three methods we may learn wisdom: first, by reflection, which is noblest; second, by imitation, which is easiest; and third by experience, which is the bitterest."

Confucius

Do you remember why you got started in smoking cigarettes? May be it was peer pressure. Perhaps you thought it was "cool" or made you look "independent," "tough," or "sophisticated." May be you started in your teens and thought that smoking would make you an "adult." Or you saw a movie star or a celebrity you like smoking. Or you were just curious. May be a combination of all of these. And the exposure to all the cool looking cigarette ads certainly did not prevent you from reaching for the smokes. Whatever the reason, you probably did not like how cigarette tasted when you took that first puff. No smoker ever does. You probably choked a little and coughed out the toxic smoke. You could not believe in your innocent mind why anyone would smoke, although you might not have expressed your true feelings to your friends. You probably wondered why anyone would choose to smoke, or thought that you could never be addicted to such a vile tasting stuff. But you persevered. It might take a couple of times, or a few. It might even take years of casual smoking or "bumming" cigarette from friends (and sometimes from strangers) before you became hooked. It takes a lot of hard work to learn how to smoke and to get to the point where you feel the urge to inhale the toxic smoke. But you have done it, and via one way or another, you have chained that nicotine beggar inside of you through your own actions.

Have you ever thought about why you keep smoking? Do you like how a cigarette tastes? I did not. Hardly any smoker actually likes the taste. That is why many smokers often spit when they are smoking. Or drink coffee, beer, or anything else while smoking to minimize the nasty taste while they get their nicotine hit. Or smoke after a meal, while your mouth and throat is coated with food to lessen the nasty cigarette taste. There's a reason why menthol cigarette (or any other type of flavoring) has a big following—the menthol (and other flavoring) masks the nasty cigarette taste. If you actually think you enjoy the taste of your cigarette, ask yourself whether you would stop smoking if your brand of cigarette was no longer available. You will find that you will simply switch to a different cigarette brand. The truth is, smokers smoke cigarettes in spite of—not because of—the cigarette taste. Smokers tolerate the rotten taste of cigarettes in order to get their "fix" of nicotine. Go ahead and light up a cigarette right now and taste it for yourself, preferably one that is not flavored with menthol or others. Feel the toxic smoke hitting your tongue, taste it, and think about if you actually enjoy it. If you are like vast majority of smokers, you will realize that cigarettes actually taste disgusting.

9   There are numerous benefits of not smoking.

"Only I can change my life. No one can do it for me."

Carol Burnett

In your quest to quit smoking, focus should be on the fact that smoking gives you no benefit. Nevertheless, you can keep the benefits of not smoking in the back of your mind. There are numerous benefits of being a nonsmoker, from physical to mental, from short term to long term, from interpersonal to global.

There are immediate physical benefits when you stop smoking. For example, your sense of smell improves and continues to improve as days go by. You stop having the "smoker's cough." You are able to breathe easier. Your lung is working as it should have been working before you started smoking. Going for a walk or taking the stairs does not leave you huffing for breath. Working out, or improving your game—whether it is basketball, tennis, golf, ultimate frisbee, or any other sports—becomes a whole lot easier.

Your taste buds come alive, as your tongue is no longer coated with nasty layers of cigarette smoke. You are now able to taste all of the subtle flavors of your favorite foods. You can now taste the freshness in fresh fruits and vegetables. You produce less phlegm. You do not cough as often, and you do not need to blow your nose as often or spit as often. Your heart rate and blood pressure begin to return to healthier level. Within few hours of stopping smoking, the level of carbon monoxide in the blood begins to decline, increasing the efficiency of your blood to carry oxygen. You no longer have bad breath. You can rid yourself of the brown and black stain in your teeth. Your circulation improves. These are just some of the many immediate physical benefits you can experience as soon as you stop smoking.

Of course, there are numerous long term health benefits of quitting smoking. As any smoker knows (at least superficially), it is undeniable that quitting smoking can add years to one's life. Smoking harms nearly every organ of the body, according to the Center for Disease Control and Prevention ("CDC"), and causes cancer in almost every part of a human body, including cancer in the mouth and throat (e.g. oropharynx, larynx, esophagus), lung, stomach, liver, pancreas, kidney, cervix, bladder, colorectal, and more. According to the Surgeon General, one out of three cancer deaths are caused by smoking. Smoking is also linked to stroke, degeneration of eyes (e.g. cataracts), orofacial clefts, teeth and gum problems (e.g. periodontitis), aneurysms, heart diseases, pneumonia, vascular diseases, tuberculosis, respiratory diseases (e.g. asthma), diabetes, fertility problems, erectile dysfunction, arthritis, and more. And of course, smoking during pregnancy risks baby's health, including premature delivery, stillbirth, low birth weight, sudden infant death syndrome, ectopic pregnancy, and other issues.

According to CDC's estimates, cigarette smoking causes more than 480,000 deaths each year just in the United States, which equates to about one in five deaths. To put the number in perspective, in the United States, smoking causes more deaths than all of the following combined: HIV, illegal drug use, alcohol use, car accidents, and gun incidents. More than 10 times as many Americans have died from cigarette smoking than those that have died in all the wars fought by the United States during its entire history. Smoking is estimated to cause about 90% of all lung cancer deaths, and about 80% of all deaths from chronic obstructive pulmonary disease (COPD). In the face of such grim statistics, some smokers like to think that they will get "lucky" and be one of the "exceptions" to the health statistics. What they do not realize is that there are no "exceptions"; smoking is already affecting their health by decreasing the lung capacity, the stamina for physical activity, and countless other ways. It is possible that you may not get lung cancer, but you will never be "lucky" if you keep smoking. Perhaps they also know of a two-packs-a day smoker who has lived until eighty years of age. But exception does not make the rule. And besides, they do not account for the possibility that the smoker might have lived a healthy life until he was a hundred years old if he had not been a smoker. Smokers may also say that they are not worried about the health because "Hey, I can get hit by a car and die tomorrow." But they are not jumping to kill themselves in a car crash, while at the same time actively risking their lives by sucking on the toxic fume that is cigarette smoke.

Smoking not only hurts the smoker's body, but also hurts innocent by-standers through secondhand smoke. Secondhand smoke causes some of the same detriment to the nonsmoker as to smokers who voluntarily choose to inhale the toxic substance. The Surgeon General estimates that living with a smoker increases a nonsmoker's chances of developing lung cancer or heart disease by 20 to 30 percent. Children exposed to secondhand smoke are at an increased risk of sudden infant death syndrome, ear infections, colds, pneumonia, bronchitis, and asthma. Secondhand smoke exposure slows the growth of children's lungs.

Quitting smoking cuts the long term health risks dramatically. For instance, your risk for a heart attack drops sharply just 1 year after quitting smoking, according to the CDC. Within 2 to 5 years after quitting smoking, your risk for stroke could fall to about the same as a nonsmoker. Risks for various cancers, including cancer of the mouth, throat, esophagus, and bladder drops by half within 5 years after quitting smoking. And your risk for lung cancer drops by half about ten years after you quit smoking. As these statistics show, it is never too late to quit smoking. You can improve your health dramatically regardless of whether you quit when you are 20 or when you are 80 (in the unlikely event that you have survived that long while being addicted to cigarettes).

Quitting smoking also fattens your wallet personally and provides economic benefits globally. The cost of a cigarette pack has gotten higher and higher over the years. A smoker's budget for cigarette can add up quickly day by day, week by week, month by month, and year by year. Think about the amount of money that you will be saving over your life time of smoking. Let's say an average pack of cigarette is $7 (in many places, it is double that amount), and let's assume that you smoke one pack per day and that you started smoking at 20 years of age and that you will smoke until 65 years of age. That means that you will have spent $114,975.00 (45 years X 365 days X $7), just so that you can suck toxic smoke, stain your teeth, make your breath smelly, and ruin your health. Imagine all of the things that you could have bought, vacations you could have taken, food that you could have enjoyed, gifts that you could have given with the money you saved feeding the nicotine beggar inside you.

The economic impact of smoking is not limited just to the costly cigarette packs you buy, but also to the increased health care costs that would inevitably result from continuing to smoke. According to the 2014 report of Surgeon General, it is estimated that smoking costs almost $300 **billion** in economic costs **annually**, with direct medical costs of at least $130 billion and productivity losses of more than $150 billion a year. The amount of resources that can be put to better use is staggering. Imagine all the hungry people you can feed with that kind of money.

Quitting smoking may also prevent interpersonal and relationship problems. For example, your friends, family and loved ones may not want you to smoke, which is entirely unsurprising given all of the detrimental effects on your health. This comes in direct conflict with your addiction, which may cause strife in your relationship. Some smokers may even promise to quit, and if the promise is not kept, that may cause further rift in a relationship. The situation could even lead to the smoker hiding his addictive behavior, lying about smoking, and other interpersonal issues. In addition, many (perhaps all) workplace discourages smoking while on the job. It is not fun being a smoker in the modern workplace. Quitting smoking eliminates all of these potential issues in personal and professional relationships, and your hair, fingers, face, clothes, and furniture will no longer have the rotten cigarette smell.

Perhaps the best part about not smoking is the benefits you get in your mental well being. You no longer need to worry about that next cigarette. You do not have to be anxious about taking a long bus/train/plane ride. You can concentrate better in long meetings or classes, without constantly thinking about when they are going to end so that you can feed your nicotine beggar. Your stress level is reduced, as you are free from the ball-and-chain of your addiction. No one needs the added stress and burden of feeding an addiction when one is already in a stressful situation, such as taking an exam, making a presentation, doing an interview, or countless other situations. All of these physical and mental benefits add up, and you will have more energy and be more "alive." It certainly is a great feeling when you realize that you do not "need" that cigarette anymore in those situations, and know that a cigarette was merely giving you added stress and irritability without any benefits.

10 When you stop smoking, you are not giving anything up.

"Be happy. It is one way of being wise." Sidonie Gabrielle Colette

There are no benefits to leave behind when you stop inhaling the cancer smoke. As such, you are not "giving anything up" when you quit smoking. It is important to truly understand this—that there are no benefits to smoking—because once you do, no willpower is needed to stop smoking. After all, you are a reasonable person, and why would a reasonable person do something that provides no benefit?

Once you have decided to stop smoking, you can rejoice in the feeling of being free from the demands of the nicotine beggar inside you. There are no advantages or benefits to smoking. As such, when faced with a trigger situation or temptation, you do not need to avoid it. Enjoy that cup of coffee. You will realize that coffee tastes a lot better without cigarettes. Cigarette merely adds nasty taste to an otherwise pleasant experience of drinking coffee. Similarly, you can enjoy the taste of your beer or cocktail, and not have the beer or cocktail serve merely as something to drown out the nasty cigarette taste. Sure, you may feel some irritation and discomfort in refraining from smoking in your "trigger" situations. People are often conditioned to believe that irritation and discomfort is "wrong" and that feeling of comfort is "right." But often times, it is ok to feel discomfort. Everyone feels a little discomfort in trying something different or meeting someone new. Without discomfort, life's most rewarding experiences will not occur. The feeling of discomfort and irritation when faced with your "trigger" situation is only natural, particularly in the first few days or weeks of your quitting. Observe your feelings, while remembering that it is the cigarette that has caused the irritability and discomfort, and that smoking will only prolong and perpetuate those feelings. Do not avoid how you feel.

Take a deep breath and remember that you have given up nothing when you quit smoking. The opposite is true. By quitting smoking, you have gained your life and freedom back. Think about it this way: By quitting smoking, you have purged a parasite inside you—the nicotine beggar—a disease of the mind and body that would have ultimately killed you. You have beat back a deadly disease. Rejoice in that fact.

11 You do not need substitutes.

"We are what our thoughts have made us; so take care about what you think. Words are secondary. Thoughts live; they travel far." Swami Vivekananda

Cigarette substitutes—such as nicotine gum, patch, e-cigarettes, and other nicotine products—may give you mixed results. Sometimes they help, but often times, such nicotine substitutes may exacerbate the nicotine addiction for obvious reasons, i.e., you are still feeding the nicotine beggar when you use a nicotine gum, patch, or similar products. Such use may make the nicotine addiction worse because one may actually consumer more nicotine than they had been consuming as a smoker! Because of such danger, it is extremely important to keep track of how much gum or patch you are using if you do decide to use them. And if you do use them, use them only for a short period of time, until you get the hang of not lighting up a smoke for those first few days. You should stop feeding the nicotine beggar as soon as you can, whether it is through cigarette smoke, through a gum, or other method. Otherwise, you will always be chained to the slavery that is nicotine addiction.

The best course of action is to not use any substitute at all. After all, you do not need a substitute for something that provides no benefits! You do not need a substitute for toxic poison. If you really feel you need a distraction in your mouth or your fingers when you feel the urge to smoke, go get some carrot sticks or celery sticks to put in your mouth or hold between your fingers. Or have a piece of gum, cough drops, or tic-tac. Or have a drink of water, take a deep breath, and feel the refreshing feeling of being free of the toxic smoke that is in a cigarette puff. And remind yourself that there are no benefits to smoking, and that you are not "giving up" anything. Soon enough, not smoking will be as natural as it was before you first took your puff of the cancer stick.

12 There is no need to reward yourself for "milestones."

"If you want to be happy, be." Leo Tolstoy

Children are often taught early on to delay gratification, and that if they do a chore or a task, they will receive some reward. People of all ages often reward themselves after finishing a dreaded task, such as treating themselves with a nice snack or meal, or a day doing their favorite fun activity. But nobody treats themselves to a reward for sitting through a movie or getting through an hour of doing their favorite hobby. Watching an hour of your favorite movie or spending an hour doing your favorite hobby is not a "milestone" that needs rewarding. That is because watching a movie or doing their favorite hobby is its own reward. Similarly, making it through one week smoke-free, or one month smoke-free, or one year smoke-free need not be rewarded, as the journey itself of being smoke-free is its own reward. You are free from the slavery that is nicotine addiction. There is no need to further reward yourself. Making a big celebration may be psychologically confusing as well, as setting such a "milestone" may make you think that you have given up something valuable to reach your "milestone." It can never be emphasized enough that you have given up nothing when you quit smoking, as smoking provides no benefits. You cleansed yourself from the dirty, needy, and toxic nicotine beggar inside you. You do not need "milestones" rewards to celebrate doing a deep cleansing of your teeth at the dentist's office. Same way, you do not need to celebrate being cleansed of the nicotine beggar for one week, one month, one year, ten years, or anything in between. You rejoice in your new found freedom day-by-day, moment-by-moment.

Being smoke-free is its own reward. Similar to the reason why "milestone" rewards are unnecessary, it is counter-productive to have a reward for stopping smoking. For example, it is counter-productive to make a bet with a friend to quit smoking, or have a loved one promise to give you a prize for quitting smoking. This is because such notion feeds the mind-trick mechanism whereby you are fooled into thinking that you are giving up something precious in exchange for the prize. It is a false incentive, a false motivation. You are not giving anything up when you are quitting smoking. You do not need to be rewarded, as you have sacrificed nothing.

13 Quitting smoking does not cause weight gain.

"You cannot wait for inspiration. You have to go after

it with a club." Jack London

Some smokers have a concern that they may gain weight if they quit smoking. This may happen if you substitute cigarette with food, which leads to overeating. If you do not overeat, you will not gain weight. The urge or the pang to smoke may often be similar to the hunger pangs that you get when you have not eaten in a while. Recognize the urges to smoke for what it is and be mindful of what you eat.

To the extent you need to have a substitute in response to your pangs, reach for a carrot or a celery stick, or sugarless gum, or just plain water. However, before you go the route of using any substitute, try to think about what you are feeling when you have the pangs. What is the sensation that you feel? Are you irritated, and if so why? When have you eaten, and are you feeling hungry for more food? Do not avoid your pangs and urges, but instead try to fully understand them. Your pangs and urges have no power over you unless you allow them to control your actions. Soon enough, your pang will subside with time even without any substitutes.

The nicotine addiction has created the situation (*i.e.* the pangs and urges) that may cause people to overeat. Do not give credit to cigarettes for keeping your weight in check. It is wholly undeserved. Your weight is entirely about the amount of food you take in and the amount of calories you burn. If you take advantage of your renewed lung capacity and exercise more, you may even lose a few pounds once you quit smoking.

14 There is no such thing as "just one drag"; do not underestimate the power of nicotine addiction.

"We are made wise not by the recollection of our past, but by the responsibility for our future." George Bernard Shaw

After you have endured the first few days, perhaps first few weeks, or even first few months, you may be presented with a tempting situation to smoke. Perhaps at a gathering with friends who smoke, or while doing one of your former "trigger" activity. The addict within you may take this opportunity to play its mind tricks again. It will tell you "just one drag," "just one puff," "just one cigarette." You might think to yourself "I can handle this," which should mean that you will not smoke. But your mind might rationalize to interpret "I can handle this" to mean "I can take just one drag and be okay; after all, it's just one puff; I'll confirm once and for all that cigarette tastes like crap and I'll really quit for good after that." You might invent other rationalization tricks to get back on your addictive behavior. But deep inside you, you know that there is no such thing as "just one puff" or "just one cigarette."

Do not think you can act on your addictive impulses without becoming an addict again. There is no "handling" of a smoke other than simply abstaining from smoking. There is no such thing as "just one drag" or "just one smoke." And your mind that is telling you such nonsense is merely playing another mind trick, and such a self-deception is created by the nicotine beggar for the sole purpose and goal of furthering the nicotine addiction. Once you fall for the "just one drag" mind trick, you will be on a familiar path—the path to enslavement again. After that "one drag," you might tell yourself that "I can handle this," which turns into "I will moderate my smoking," which turns into "I only smoke when I see my smoker friends" to "Only on weekends" to "No more than three a day," and on it goes until you are back at it again like it never stopped. The nicotine beggar will come back alive, ready to enslave you as you had been before. Do not fall for the trick of thinking that "just one drag" will be ok. Remember cigarette tastes like crap and that there are no benefits to smoking.

Moderating your cigarette intake is a dangerous and ineffective for some of the same reason as the mind trick of "just one drag." Cutting down the number of cigarettes you smoke will only make you a more miserable smoker. Let's say that you go from smoking a pack a day to two cigarettes a day. Now, instead of being in withdrawal 30 minutes at a time, you will be in withdrawal 5-10 hours at a time. Your day will revolve around those two cigarettes, and when you can have those "precious" cigarettes. Your mind will fool yourself into thinking cigarettes as the most precious and dear thing in the world. That is how a human mind works—if one is deprived of something, one longs for and is led to believe that that thing is desirable. As such, cutting down is likely to make it harder for you to quit. As long as you keep smoking, your withdrawal symptoms will never stop and be perpetuated day by day. Stopping completely is the only way to become a nonsmoker. Cutting down or the mindset of "I'm moderating it" will not work.

If you really think you can handle it, then handle it by not smoking. The only way to quit smoking for good is to stop engaging in addictive behavior, such as "just one drag." Do not give into rationalizations and complications, which are merely mind tricks invented by your nicotine-conditioned brain. Do not give in to "just one drag." Quitting smoking is not easy, but it is a simple process—simple in that the only thing you need to do is to stop smoking. Anything more complicated is just mind tricks attempting to trick you into the path back to the nicotine addiction.

15 Be free from the deadly disease that is addiction to smoking.

"For what avail the plough or sale,

Or land or life, if freedom fail?"

Ralph Waldo Emerson

Your state of mind and perspective is everything. After all, your mind is how you see, feel, and understand the world. So it is with your addiction to cigarettes. I hope you have convinced yourself that cigarettes provide no benefit to you, and that you are able to recognize the mind tricks that your nicotine beggar creates in your brain for what they are—tricks to get you to feed the addiction. If you truly understand this—that smoking has no value or advantage— you will have no problem stopping smoking. You will be happy, as you should, that you have ridden yourself of a deadly disease inside you. Think of how great it is to not be enslaved by nicotine stick that takes your health little-by-little without giving anything back to you. When you are putting out that last cigarette of your life, you are stamping out a life of slavery, tension, and stress, and starting a new life of freedom, peace, and vigor. Now, if you have not already done so, throw out all the cigarettes that you have. You have made the decision to quit, so you do not need cigarettes lying around to create any doubt. Have no doubt in your mind that you will smoke no more.

It does not require willpower to quit. All you need to do is to understand the fact that smoking provides no benefit. You are not giving up anything when you quit smoking. Just remember that fact whenever you have the "urge," and be happy about your choice not to smoke. Be wary of your mind's tendency to try to make things more complicated, as complication is a sign that the nicotine beggar is conjuring up mind tricks. Quitting smoking is a simple process: You make the decision to stop smoking, and you happily stop smoking. You can do this!